Books is an imprint of Summersdale Publishers Ltd

Summersdale Publishers Ltd
West Street
Chichester
West Sussex
PO19 1RP

www.summersdale.com

Printed and bound in the Czech Republic

ISBN: 978-1-84953-578-6

Substantial discounts on bulk quantities of Summersdale books are available to corporations, professional associations and other organisations. For details contact Nicky Douglas by telephone: +44 (0) 1243 756902, fax: +44 (0) 1243 786300, or email: nicky@summersdale.com.

50 TIPS
TO HELP YOU THROUG
MENOPAU

C
T
tr
in
a
in

Vi

Su
46
CH
We
PO
UK

ww

Prin

ISBN

Subs
are
orga
+44
nicky

50 TIPS
TO HELP YOU THROUGH THE
MENOPAUSE

Anna Barnes

Introduction

Myriad changes take place in the body during menopause, and most women find the best solution is to embrace the change and create something positive. The menopause can affect women in a variety of ways and you may find that your symptoms and experiences differ from those of others, but there are many safe and natural ways to combat them, such as adapting your diet and lifestyle, incorporating exercise and mindfulness into your daily routine, and generally dropping bad habits you'd be better off without. These easy-to-follow tips offer ways in which you can make this experience easier to manage. However, if at any point you find the menopause is causing you too much difficulty, you should seek advice from your GP.

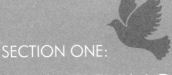

SECTION ONE:

IDENTIFYING THE MENOPAUSE

Every woman with ovaries will experience the menopause as she approaches middle age. Whichever survival techniques you choose to employ, you might first find it helpful to understand what is happening and why.

Understand the menopause

The menopause is the end of menstruation, when a woman experiences her last period, and her body stops producing the hormones oestrogen and progesterone. Each woman's ovaries carry a limited supply of eggs and when these run out, and are no longer released each month, periods stop. The dip in hormone levels causes changes to occur in the body. Menopause usually occurs between the ages of 45 and 55, and the average age in the UK is 52. In rare cases, menopause occurs before the age of 45, sometimes as early as in the

20s or 30s – this is called early menopause and usually requires overseeing by a GP as, in addition to its impact on fertility, it can also have long-term consequences for heart and bone health. Every woman will reach the menopause, but each will experience different symptoms; a lucky few will experience none at all.

Identify the symptoms

The changes that come with menopause are varied and unpredictable, and individual to each woman; it is important to remember, however, that it is a normal, natural process. The first sign is that your periods may become more frequent or infrequent. Whatever the scenario, it's worth heading to your GP for a reassuring chat and having your hormone levels checked by a simple blood test. Although experts advise women to continue using contraception for a year after their last period, as there is still a chance they could fall pregnant. Any bleeding 12 months after the date of your last period also warrants a trip to the GP. The most common complaints from women reaching menopause include hot flushes and night sweats, loss of libido, changes in mood, anxiety, depression, insomnia, vaginal dryness and urinary tract infections. But don't despair – many women find this is a time in their life in which to embrace change and improve their lifestyle; whether you choose to do this by adapting your diet, or incorporating exercise or holistic approaches into your routine.

Top up with hormone replacement therapy

Hormone replacement therapy (HRT) is the medication commonly prescribed by GPs to women who have either reached the menopause or are at the perimenopausal stage (the years leading up to the menopause). HRT replaces the oestrogen hormones women's bodies have been used to receiving since puberty, which cease production once they reach the menopause. The 'topping up' of oestrogen levels can help to make you feel more your usual self as your body goes through changes. There are plenty of complementary therapies that you could try before opting for HRT and many women choose to take the natural route, and replace the lost oestrogen by incorporating foods into their diet that are rich in phytoestrogens – plant hormones that have a similar effect on the body as oestrogen. (See also the chapter on 'How Your Diet Can Help' to find out which foods contain phytoestrogens.) HRT is also often used to treat early menopause to help reduce the risk of more serious health consequences (e.g. osteoporosis and heart disease).

4

Keep a diary

It might be an idea to start keeping a diary of your symptoms in order to keep track of the changes happening to your body. Try to keep a log of any unusual emotions you may be experiencing or any physical changes you are noticing – just brief notes or lists will do. You may find this beneficial if you need to look back and assess your progress, and if you decide to seek medical help it will be useful to have kept a record. It may also assist you in finding out which of the following tips work best, whether it's complementary therapies, incorporating certain vitamins and minerals into your diet, or embracing a new form of exercise.

SECTION TWO:

HOW TO COPE WITH THE HEAT

It's common to experience hot flushes when you reach the menopause, but don't despair — try these tips to stay cool and calm if and when they do occur.

Learn to spot the signs

Hot flushes are most common in the year that follows your final period and eight out of ten menopausal women in the UK claim to have experienced them. Women at the perimenopausal stage have also been known to experience hot flushes, although this is not as common. You may notice a feeling of heat spreading across your upper body, often starting around the face, neck or chest, before moving upwards or downwards. You may find the affected areas become red and patchy, your heart rate increases, and you feel dizzy and may break into a sweat. The best way to beat the heat is to be prepared; this will not only help to cool you down when the hot flush does occur, but will keep you calm knowing that you have things under control and are ready for anything. There are several factors that may cause you to experience a hot flush, which you will learn to avoid. It might be an idea to reduce your caffeine and alcohol intake, as these have been found to trigger hot flushes. Spicy food is also a known trigger, as it can raise your body temperature, so avoid those scorching curries and instead opt for soya-rich products, chickpeas, and plenty of fruit and veg.

6

Choose your clothes wisely

One way to prepare for any unwanted heat surges is to be aware of your clothing. In the warmer months, opt for cotton or linen fabrics (the higher percentage the better), which allows your skin to breathe, rather than synthetic (polyester, acrylic, nylon, etc.). Make sure your clothes are not too restrictive, as this may cause you to feel uncomfortable. This doesn't mean you have to wear a loose-fitting sack – it is still perfectly possible to look stylish and feel comfortable at the same time. In the colder months, try wearing several thin layers instead of a bulky woolly jumper, as these can be removed discreetly in the event that you need to cool down quickly.

Keep your handbag handy

You may find it's useful to carry a few essential 'tools' as you go about your daily routine, just in case a hot flush is imminent. Keep a small water spray bottle with you to help you cool down; you could either spray this on the insides of your wrists, or lightly onto your face – although you may then also need to touch up make-up, if you wear it. Wet wipes may be useful to have with you, along with tissues, and a pocket fan is also a good idea for a quick cool-down fix. It's also important to drink enough water. Carry a small bottle with you, and sip it little and often to keep your hydration levels up. This will help you keep cool, as well as supporting healthy brain function, which will help you stay alert and calm.

8

Keep a fan nearby

As well as carrying a pocket fan in your handbag, it might be useful to set up a larger model at home or work to help you to keep cool. If you work in an office environment, a desk fan is unlikely to bother anyone else — ask if they mind first, and if they do, at least you can use your pocket version. You might also find it soothing to set up a fan in your bedroom, especially during the warmer months, in order to help combat any night sweats you may be experiencing and keep air flowing through the room during the night.

SECTION THREE:

BOOST YOUR MOOD

Some women find themselves experiencing bouts of low mood and anxiety during the menopause. Use these tips to reach for a more positive outlook.

9

Understand your mood

The changes in your mood are due to the dip in hormones experienced during menopause. Your ovaries are no longer producing oestrogen, and this can lead to you feeling emotionally unbalanced. You've also reached a point in your life where you can no longer have children. Perhaps you have them already or perhaps you don't; perhaps you never wanted them. Whatever the case, you may experience emotions about the finality of this life change. The menopause is something of a life marker, signalling the next phase. Try to focus on the good points of being at the stage you are in life; take time to look back at all that you have achieved so far, be it a family you are proud of, your career, home life or network of friends. Weigh up the positive and not so positive aspects of your life and make a pact with yourself to do what you can to combat the latter.

10

De-stress yourself

Many menopausal women experience increased levels of stress at this point of their lives. This is generally due to hormonal changes, and disrupted sleep patterns and hot flushes are likely to only exacerbate things. A good way to relieve stress is to remove it from your surroundings. If you look around your home and feel overwhelmed by the number of chores you have to carry out, take things one step at a time and create a list of tasks you can cross off as you come to each one. This will help you feel a sense of achievement and progress. Decluttering can be particularly cathartic, while creating more space in the home can help to bring a sense of calm. Clear out and organise your wardrobe to make your mornings less stressful, and make sure everything has a place in your home. If you're finding financial worries are getting on top of you, create a spreadsheet and make sense of your monthly outgoings – are there areas where you could cut down on your spending? If you're finding work too stressful, learn to say 'no' and delegate tasks to others when you have too much on; create a pleasant work environment by replacing mess with calming influences, such as plants or photographs.

Beat the blues

It's common for women who have reached the menopause to experience bouts of depression and anxiety – you're not alone and there are plenty of simple steps you can take to help combat these feelings. While it's perfectly natural to feel down, many women look to the menopause as a positive time in their lives when they can change their lifestyle for the better and never look back. Perhaps now is the time to adapt your diet and experiment with a new exercise regime. A healthy combination of good diet and regular exercise can work wonders to boost your mood and could help you on the path to becoming healthier and happier. And look on the bright side – no more periods!

12

Boost your mood with exercise

If you're feeling anxious or stressed, or are suffering from the dreaded hot flushes, working out may be the furthest thing from your mind. But getting regular exercise is proven to help boost your mood, as well as relieve stress, and is a sure-fire way to get you on the path to positivity. Exercise promotes the release of endorphins, which are the body's natural painkillers and make us feel good. Talk of the 'runner's high' refers to the surge of endorphins released when an athlete reaches a certain point in a race or in their routine, with some claiming to have felt a sense of euphoria and a feeling of peace. Try it and see how it works for you.

13

Find a support network

Remember, as you reach the menopause, that you are not alone and there are plenty of people who will understand what you're going through. The Internet is a wonderful tool – visit www.menopausematters.co.uk to learn more about this stage of your life and discover a wealth of information, as well as forums where like-minded women are discussing various issues. If you feel you need more human contact in your support network, look for groups that meet up locally to talk through their experiences; for those who have gone through early menopause, www.daisynetwork.org.uk is a registered charity specialising in offering help and advice, as well as forums and information on support groups. Friends and family will also be more than happy to lend an ear, and vocalising your issues will no doubt help to lift a weight from your shoulders.

14

Make time for sex

Many women experiencing the menopause find their libido is significantly diminished, as oestrogen plays a vital part in heightening sex drive and the menopausal hormone imbalance can affect this. Women tend to reach their sexual peak in their late 30s and 40s, so a sudden loss of libido can be somewhat disconcerting. You may also experience dryness, where the skin of the vaginal walls thins making sex painful, but there are moisturisers and lubricants that can help. You may find taking a gentle, relaxed approach is the way forward. There are many who believe it's all about attitude and that, with the right one, your sex life can in fact flourish as you enter the next phase of your life. Refer to websites such as www.menopausematters.co.uk and www.menopause.org for helpful advice.

15

Think positively

Although it's often easier said than done, it's important to make an effort to stay as positive as possible when you're prone to experiencing low mood. Try not to let your symptoms overwhelm you and focus on the changes you can make to combat them. Keep active and busy, focus on your work, and meet regularly with family and friends. Talk to others who share similar symptoms and share tips on how to stay on top of things. Keeping those negative thoughts at bay will have a positive impact on your life as a whole. (See also the chapters on 'How Your Diet Can Help' and 'Try Supplements' to understand more about boosting your mood.)

16

Try a little laughter therapy

Our muscles tend to relax when we laugh, and those feel-good endorphins are released into our bloodstream. So, if you're feeling low, laughter therapy might be worth a try. It's a great form of therapy and will no doubt leave you feeling better. Try standing in an empty room and forcing yourself to laugh – you might feel silly, but it can work wonders. Take things one step further and get some friends together for a laughter therapy session. Sit in a circle and take turns to start. The first person should say 'ha', the second 'ha ha', the third 'ha ha ha' and so on until everyone dissolves into laughter.

17

Get out in the sun

We might be prone to drizzly, grey days in the UK – which doesn't help matters when we're experiencing low mood – but when the sun does come out it's important to take advantage of the goodness it can offer us. Our bodies create most of our vitamin D from direct sunlight and this helps the brain to produce serotonin, our 'happy hormone'. Fewer hours of sunlight in the winter months can lead us to feel sleepier than usual, as when it is dark our brains produce melatonin, the 'sleep hormone'. Experts have found that brief, daily periods of direct sunlight – around ten to fifteen minutes – can give us the vitamin D we need to pep us up; after this you should apply sun cream to avoid any sun damage. Even on cloudy days we can still reap the benefits, although it takes our bodies a little longer to produce the vitamin D.

SECTION FOUR:
EMBRACE EXERCISE

Getting regular exercise is a great way to build a positive outlook. Try these simple tips to incorporate more activity into your daily routine.

18

Get active

During exercise, the body releases serotonin, the 'happy hormone', which is naturally great for boosting your mood. Being more active will also improve your fitness level, tone your muscles, increase your positivity by making you feel more confident, and help you to sleep better. These days, more of us work longer hours than ever before, and it's easy to let the week go by without seeing much in the way of daylight or doing much physical activity other than walking to and from the car, train station or bus stop. If you're struggling to fit in exercise, why not get off the bus a few stops earlier and walk the rest of the way? Or leave the car at home if you only need to make a short trip.

Swim for it

Swimming is a great form of exercise and offers myriad health benefits – both physically and psychologically. As well as helping to tone and strengthen muscles, increase your flexibility and help keep your heart healthy, spending half an hour in the pool will instil a sense of calm and give you a more positive outlook, making you feel good about yourself and your body. Give your local swimming pool a chance and, if it works for you, think about signing up for a membership so you will be inclined to go for a dip more often. Try and fit in a swim at lunchtime or before or after work, and incorporate it into your routine.

Get on your bike

Fresh air and exercise are a good combination to help raise positivity and fitness levels, especially if you're feeling the menopause taking its toll. As well as being an efficient mode of transport, cycling is also an enjoyable way to get regular exercise and de-stress while enjoying the scenery. If you currently drive to work, or use public transport, and the distance is manageable, think about cycling instead. If you'd rather take the scenic route, visit the Sustrans website, www.sustrans.org.uk, and learn about the cycling routes in your area.

The UK National Cycle Network comprises 14,000 miles of safe traffic-free paths and quiet road routes throughout the country. Sustrans claims a safe NCN route passes within a mile of 55 per cent of UK homes. There could be a wealth of green space on the outskirts of your home town, just waiting to be explored, so get on your bike and ride your way to a happier you.

21

Take a walk in the park

If cycling doesn't appeal, walking is a great, easy way to get fresh air and sunshine while boosting your mood and instilling a sense of calm, and it doesn't cost a penny. If you live close to, or in the heart of, the countryside then you have no excuse – get out there and enjoy your surroundings! Alternatively, why not drive or use public transport to take you to some nearby green spaces and take in a loop walk or pick up a bus when you get to the end. Visit www.nationaltrail.co.uk

or www.nationaltrust.org.uk to find suitable walking routes in your area. You could also make a conscious effort to walk more day to day, rather than drive or use public transport and always take the stairs instead of using the lift – these small bursts of exercise all add up, after all, and will go some way to help you to feel less sluggish and more alert.

SECTION FIVE:

HOW YOUR DIET CAN HELP

Making a few changes to your daily diet can have a positive impact on both your physical and psychological symptoms. Consider these dietary tips and see how they work for you.

Know your fats

Research has found that those who diet and cut out all types of fat can experience feelings of anxiety and depression, so when going through the menopause you need to incorporate the good types of fat into your diet in order to retain a positive outlook. Not all fats are bad news. Of the four types of fat, the unhealthy varieties, saturated and trans fats, should be avoided or consumed in moderation. However, polyunsaturated fats are vital to healthy brain functioning, while monounsaturated fats are rich in vitamin E, and both can help to lower cholesterol. The former can be found in walnuts, peanuts, sesame and sunflower seeds, olive oil and oily fish; while the latter can be found in red meat, full-fat milk, nuts, olives and avocados — so incorporate these foods into your daily diet if you can. It might also be an idea to stick to lean protein and reduce your sugar intake.

23

Up your fruit and veg intake

The recommended daily intake of fruit and vegetables in the UK is five portions – are you getting your five a day? As well as contributing to your general wellbeing, certain fruits and vegetables can also help to reduce menopausal symptoms. Opt for green leafy vegetables (think broccoli, cabbage, kale and Brussels sprouts), as well as green and red peppers, courgettes, carrots and French beans – as these contain phytoestrogens, the plant hormone that can help to do the same job as oestrogen in the human body. Green vegetables also contain glucosinolates, which are believed to protect against breast cancer. So incorporate as many of these into your diet as you can; the fresher the better – try a stir-fry with a pile of the above vegetables, lightly cooked so they remain crunchy and retain as much of their goodness as possible. Cranberries play an important role in protecting against and treating urinary tract infections, so try and incorporate a glass of cranberry juice a day into your routine too.

24

Watch what's on your plate

It's important to eat regularly, even if you have a hectic schedule, as this will help to keep mood swings at bay. Three meals a day is essential; eat them at evenly spaced intervals and this will help to maintain your blood sugar levels. As tempting as it may be to skip breakfast, don't! Missing the first meal of the day will cause a dip in your blood sugar, which can lead to low mood. If you find yourself feeling hungry and somewhat irritable in between your three regular meals, grab a banana or a similarly healthy snack, such as a handful of nuts or some rice cakes, to keep you going until your next meal is due.

Believe in boron

Research has found that foods rich in the mineral boron can be beneficial to women experiencing menopausal symptoms, as it can help to increase oestrogen levels, in some cases to levels as high as those experienced through hormone replacement therapy. Foods containing boron include kidney beans, chickpeas, lentils, olives, vegetables (particularly green vegetables, broccoli, carrots, celery and potatoes), fruit (particularly apples, apricots, avocadoes, bananas, dates, red grapes, oranges, peaches, pears, prunes and raisins) and nuts (particularly almonds, Brazil nuts, cashews, hazelnuts and walnuts). Nuts, including peanuts, are also particularly good sources of boron, so indulge in a slice of peanut butter on toast every now and again.

26

Feed your skin

Many women complain of suffering from dry skin as they reach the menopause and there are foods you can incorporate into your diet that can help. Nuts and seeds can be good sources of vitamin E, zinc and calcium, which can help prevent dry skin as well as aiding in the normalising of hormone levels. Try almonds, and sunflower and pumpkin seeds in particular. Snack on a handful of these nuts and seeds each day or sprinkle them on salads; or, alternatively, use a coffee grinder to reduce the seeds to a fine powder, keep in an airtight container and add a heaped spoonful to soups and stews while cooking – a particularly good way to obtain the nutrients if you're not the world's biggest seed fan.

Plump for phytoestrogens

Foods that contain the plant oestrogen phytoestrogen can play a role in helping to balance your hormones. Your body may no longer be producing oestrogen, but your body has the ability to convert phytoestrogens into a substance that provides similar benefits. Phytoestrogens are found mainly in cereals, beansprouts, soya products, chickpeas, sweet potatoes, garlic, flaxseed, most nuts, and dried prunes, apricots and dates. Incorporating some of these foods into your diet may help to improve the hormone imbalance you experience when you reach the menopause, and in turn ease your symptoms and promote healthy mental wellbeing. Try adding nuts to your snacking routine and sprinkle dried fruits on desserts.

Understand vitamins and minerals

The hormone oestrogen promotes the absorption of calcium into the bones, so when your body stops producing it you may need a helping hand from elsewhere. When oestrogen stops assisting bone renewal, the risk of osteoporosis increases. Foods rich in phytoestrogens will assist as they release a substance which has a similar effect on the body, but you may also want to incorporate more calcium into your diet. This vital mineral can be obtained from milk and dairy foods, green, leafy vegetables (such as broccoli and cabbage), nuts, and soya beans and products (e.g. tofu). It's also important to make sure that you're consuming enough major vitamins, as research has found that vitamin C (found in oranges, strawberries, red and green peppers, broccoli and potatoes) and vitamin E (found in nuts, seeds, cereals and avocados) can go some way to reducing hot flushes and can help with vaginal dryness. Vitamin C is also useful for protecting against urinary tract infections and boosting your immune system, while vitamin E is very good for problem dry skin, which can occur during menopause. The ideal is to try to incorporate as many of these foods as possible into your dietary routine, but if you feel you're not getting enough of what you need, you could consider taking a supplement.

Cut down on caffeine

If you're a real caffeine junkie, you might find cutting down has a positive effect on your menopausal symptoms. Many women cite caffeine as being the trigger for hot flushes and find removing it from their diets leads to a reduction in the dreaded bouts of overheating. Caffeine is a stimulant, which increases mental and physical functioning, so if you're feeling at all anxious it will increase those feelings and could leave you feeling jittery. The amount of caffeine in a cup of tea or coffee varies according to the strength of the brand, the amount you use and brewing time, so be aware of these factors if you absolutely can't forego your morning cup of Joe.

Bloom with St John's wort

If you're experiencing bouts of low mood, St John's wort is a natural antidepressant, which many have found to be an effective short-term treatment for their depression or anxiety. Many SAD (seasonal affective disorder) sufferers choose to take St John's wort throughout the winter months, when they might not be getting as much sunlight, and therefore producing insufficient serotonin (the 'happy hormone'). This perennial yellow flowering herb has been used to treat emotional disorders for thousands of years and studies have found it to be effective in treating bouts of mild to moderate depression. You could try the one-a-day tablets, available from most pharmacists and health shops, or alternatively the herbal tea, which tends to be cheaper and has been deemed just as effective.

Assess your alcohol intake

Some women also find that alcohol can trigger hot flushes, so you may want to reduce your intake and see how it affects your symptoms. Unwinding with a glass of wine after a long day or enjoying a drink with a meal is, for some, one of life's small pleasures, so don't feel you have to cut it out completely, but if alcohol turns out to one of your triggers then you may find you'd rather cut down than suffer the consequences. Alcohol is also a depressant and tends to alter or exaggerate your current state of mind, so if you're experiencing low mood this may be another good reason to curb your intake. Certain red wines, on the other hand, can have a positive effect on those who are sleep deprived, so if you fancy a glass of wine in the evening, consider opting for red. Grape skins, which are removed during the production of white wines but left on for red, contain the sleep hormone melatonin, so a small glass before bed can work wonders. Merlot and Cabernet Sauvignon grapes have been found to be particularly rich in melatonin.

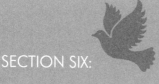

SECTION SIX:

TRY SUPPLEMENTS

There are several oft-relied-on herbal remedies and supplements that could help ease your menopausal symptoms. Always check with your GP first if you're taking any other form of medication.

32

Go-to evening primrose oil

Evening primrose oil can be beneficial to women during various stages of their reproductive life, having been found effective in the treatment of premenstrual tension (PMT) and cramps. Research has also found it to be beneficial in alleviating inflammation of the joints in those suffering from arthritis, helpful for skin conditions (such as psoriasis and eczema) and it has been known to lower cholesterol too. It is the go-to supplement for women as they reach the menopause, as it is widely recognised for its ability to reduce the occurrence of hot flushes, particularly night sweats. You may need to take evening primrose oil daily, for up to three months, before you notice the benefits, so don't give up – a little perseverance could go a long way to improving your symptoms.

33

Care for your bones with calcium

A lack of oestrogen can affect the absorption of calcium into the bones and put you at higher risk of bone weakness and osteoporosis, so it's important to make sure you are getting enough of this essential mineral. (See also the chapter on 'How Your Diet Can Help' for other helpful vitamins and minerals.) There are various foods you can incorporate more of into your diet (think broccoli and other green, leafy vegetables, soya beans, milk, cheese and other dairy products, nuts, tofu and small fish – if you eat the bones), but if you feel you need an extra top up of calcium, you might want to take a supplement. You can find various calcium supplements on your local high street, available in tablet or liquid form, as well as combination tablets that may well offer another vitamin or mineral you feel you might need.

Balance hormones with black cohosh and agnus castus

A member of the buttercup family, the perennial herb black cohosh grows largely in North America and has been used for centuries by Native Americans to treat gynaecological problems. Its oestrogenic properties have made it a useful supplement for many menopausal women, and it has been found to be effective in reducing the occurrence of hot flushes and depression in particular. Available in a tablet, capsule or liquid extract, if you're taking any other medication or suffer from liver problems, it's worth checking with your GP before you start taking black cohosh, and that goes for any of these supplements; they might all hail from natural sources and be available over the counter in health food shops, but that doesn't mean they can't react with medication and it's always better to be safe. The herb agnus castus can also be used to balance hormone levels, and many women find it helpful in reducing mood swings, anxiety and tension during menopause.

35

Add a little flaxseed

Research has found that flaxseed can be beneficial to women suffering from hot flushes and night sweats. The seed contains phytoestrogen, the plant hormone that has a similar effect on the body as oestrogen, and can therefore help to keep your hormones better balanced. Studies have shown that women who consumed a teaspoon of ground flaxseed a day found a reduction in their sudden bouts of overheating and also reported a boost in their mood. Flaxseed also contains omega-3, which has a positive effect on heart and bone health. So why not buy a large bag of flaxseed, reduce to a fine powder in a coffee grinder (this ensures the absorption of the goodness into your body) and, once a day, add a heaped teaspoon to one of your meals. The powder will disappear into soups, stews and pasta sauces, and you'll forget you're even consuming it until you start to notice the positive effects.

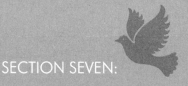

SECTION SEVEN:

HOW TO SLEEP SOUNDLY

Women who have reached the menopause find they suffer from bouts of insomnia. Whether it's night sweats or anxiety keeping you from slumber, try these suggestions for a good night's kip.

36

Make your bedroom enticing

Most adults find their optimum sleep time lies between seven to nine hours a night – work out yours and try and stick to it. Do everything you can to switch off before you go to bed. Make your bedroom a sanctuary – a place for sleep and sex only; keep it tidy, with floors clear, and find a home somewhere else in the house for everything that doesn't naturally belong there. Doing this will help you to leave daily life in another room as you prepare for sleep.

Remove any tablets, phones and laptops, and try reading a magazine or a book instead of watching TV. You may also want to opt for soft side-lighting, to give the room a warm glow, and try scented candles or oils to further create a relaxing and pleasant atmosphere. Try lavender, chamomile, jasmine or vanilla – all believed to help promote sleep.

37

Clear your mind

Many insomnia sufferers claim that their inability to get a good night's sleep is due to an overactive mind, so it's important to learn to pack up your worries before you head off to bed. Write down how you're feeling and see if this helps to unburden your mind – perhaps you could write a diary or make a to-do list for the next day; the aim is to feel as stress-free as possible before your head hits the pillow. Have a bath using some essential oils, but nothing too overpowering, to help you wind down, and have a cup of herbal tea – something containing lavender, chamomile, vanilla, hops or valerian, all natural sleep inducers.

Keep cool

Many women experience night sweats when they reach the menopause, which disrupt their sleeping patterns. You might find that one minute you are very hot, so you remove any excess layers, but the next you are very cold. Try and keep your bedroom as cool as possible; during the warmer months open the windows in the evening to allow air to flow through your bedroom and, if you feel the need, set up a fan nearby for when you feel as if you are overheating. During the winter months try and keep the radiators turned down low in the room in which you sleep. Wear cotton nightwear to allow your skin to breathe and keep a glass of water nearby, so you can take regular sips and cool down throughout the night without having to get out of bed.

Create a screen-free zone

Experts have found that spending too much time in front of backlit devices, such as the TV, computer or laptop, tablet or mobile phone, can have a detrimental effect on our ability to get to sleep, as bright screens can cause our brain to 'wake up'. Two or more hours of exposure to any of the above devices has been found to suppress melatonin, the sleep hormone, and so clearly hinders sleep. If you can take a break from any screens before bedtime you are likely to reap the sleep-laden benefits. Try removing all backlit devices from your bedroom and using a good old-fashioned alarm clock instead of your phone, as this may help you to avoid the temptation to tweet, text or email just before bed.

40

Choose the right sheets

The fabric your bed linen is made from could be the key to keeping you cool when experiencing night sweats. Opt for natural fibres, such as unbleached cotton, as these will allow your skin to breathe. Bed sheets don't have to be expensive – Egyptian cotton may be the best quality available, but a cotton or percale blend will be more affordable and will still allow you to sleep in comfort. Linen sheets also promote ventilation and have a natural cooling effect, but are on the pricier side. You may also want to use a summer-weight duvet, even in the winter, if you're feeling the heat and finding it difficult to obtain restful sleep.

41

Give lavender a go

Lavender is known in aromatherapy for its soothing and medicinal properties, and it has also been found to help induce relaxation and sleep. You could try adding a few drops of lavender oil to a pre-bed bath or drinking a lavender-infused herbal tea to help you drop off. A lavender-filled pillow left on your bed throughout the day will also leave a pleasant aroma, which you may find helps. You could also invest in a pillow mist, if you prefer the scent to be a little stronger, or put a few lavender plants on your windowsill to help fill your bedroom with the relaxing fragrance.

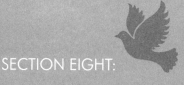

SECTION EIGHT:

TIME OUT AND TREATMENT

As you enter this new phase of your life, it's important to find time for yourself and learn how to relax fully, as well as finding the natural treatments that suit you best – try these tips and see what works for you.

Indulge in a little 'me' time

If you're finding the menopause is leaving you prone to low moods, try and make time for yourself, away from the stresses and strains of work and daily life. When there's a lot going on, it's important to have time to yourself to relax and gather your thoughts – or simply forget all about them. Perhaps you could spend an evening curled up with a good book or your favourite film, or take yourself off for a scenic walk, or simply find the time to do something you enjoy and appreciate your own company. Even going for a run or a swim – usually solitary forms of exercise – will give you a chance to think about your day while doing something that will have a positive effect on your body and mind.

Take regular breaks from work

Whatever your job, it's vital to take regular breaks from work and spend time doing what makes you happy. Whether you go on holiday or stay at home, you need time away from your daily routine to relax and switch off, and just forget about it all for a week or a few days. The 'staycation' has become ever more popular – so if you don't like travelling or don't want to break the bank, there's nothing wrong with staying close to home, as long as you do something different. Many people take time off to get things done that they wouldn't usually have time for – such as odd jobs around the house and catching up with friends.

44

Try a day of relaxation

A real treat to send your body and mind to new heights of bliss and relaxation is a spa day or weekend, where there is little to do but swim, sit in a sauna or hot tub, and enjoy de-stressing treatments, such as an aromatherapy massage or facial. This needn't be expensive – there are plenty of daily deals and dedicated websites offering discounted spa experiences, and it's likely you'll be able to find one not too far away. Keep an eye on www.groupon.com, www.livingsocial.com, www.lastminute.com and www.spabreaks.com for special offers, and arrange to get away from it all for a day or two. Either take yourself to a spa armed with a good book or magazine, or invite a friend or two to spend the experience with you, and enjoy the delightful combination of good company and relaxation.

Embrace essential oils and massage

Massage is a great way to relieve any physical tension you might be feeling and will have a calming effect on your mind too. You could opt for a professional massage or ask your partner to help. There are a range of essential oils thought to be beneficial to those experiencing menopause, so it's worth adding one or two of these to your favourite massage oil. Cypress, geranium, lavender, neroli, rose and clary sage are all thought to go some way to help balance hormones; while clary sage, flaxseed, lemon and peppermint have been found to help ease the severity of hot flushes and night sweats; and chamomile, bergamot, jasmine and neroli can help ease emotional stress and anxiety with their calming and uplifting qualities. Alternatively, you could dab a little onto your wrists or behind your ears, so the scent stays with you, and this may help keep you relaxed throughout your day.

46

Say, 'yes please' to yoga

Designed to improve back posture, strengthen muscles and increase flexibility, yoga also aims to help clear your mind and instil a sense of calm, and has been found to be extremely helpful in alleviating stress and anxiety, which many women experience during menopause. Yoga is widely practised and you're likely to find several options available locally. It can be practised in several different forms, so it's worth doing a little research to find out which is right for you. Hatha yoga is a gentle form of exercise that involves moving the body into, and holding, various postures, all the while maintaining slow, regular breathing, and is considered the best form if you're a beginner; Iyengar yoga is similarly gentle and recommended for the less active; while physically demanding ashtanga yoga comprises a series of repetitive, flowing poses, helping to build strength and synchronise breathing; and Bikram yoga is very active and demanding, and is practised in a hot room to promote sweating, and thus the clearance of toxins from the body.

Re-energise with acupuncture

Traditional acupuncture is a branch of Chinese medicine dating back some two thousand years, whereby various physical and psychological conditions are treated through the practice of pricking the skin with small needles in order to stimulate certain points on the body – thus helping to correct any imbalance to the flow of qi (natural energy). Acupuncture treatment has been found to help with both hot flushes and mood swings in women who have reached menopause. Acupuncture is recognised by the NHS as a viable treatment for certain conditions, although referral via your GP is required. Visit the British Acupuncture Council website, www.acupuncture.org.uk, to find a practising acupuncturist in your area and see if it works for you.

Practise Pilates

Pilates, as well as yoga, has been found to be beneficial to those suffering from sleep issues, helping them to find a sense of calm at bedtime, and is a good activity if you're looking to take some time out for yourself. Pilates is a low-impact, mindful form of exercise designed to strengthen the abdominal muscles, while promoting good posture, and lengthening and strengthening all the muscles in the body. Pilates has been found to have a positive effect on mood through its encouragement of deep, controlled breathing. Visit www.pilatesfoundation.com to learn more and to find a teacher in your local area. If there isn't a teacher nearby, you could buy a DVD and learn from that, or try watching some videos on YouTube.

Be mindful

Practising mindfulness, which has its origins in the Buddhist tradition, can be helpful in reducing any stress and anxiety you're feeling due to the menopause; focusing on the present encourages you to simply be at peace with yourself and live in the moment. You can practise mindfulness through meditation or introduce it into familiar situations throughout your day. For example, if you take the dog for a walk in the morning, don't go into autopilot mode and let your mind wander to other things, but instead focus on your surroundings – fill your lungs with fresh air and take in the scenery – how does it make you feel? Meditation is another good way to relax if you are feeling the need to escape the stresses of daily life, as it can help train your mind to focus and be still. Find a class or a teacher locally and see what meditation can do for you; www.1meditation.co.uk offers classes in five UK locations, but there are likely to be several options available to you if one of those doesn't happen to suit.

50

Know help is always at hand

If you're struggling with the menopause, it might be reassuring to know that many women find complementary therapies, a new exercise routine and an improved diet can work wonders. Knowing which foods can boost your mood and help balance your hormones is vital to improving your situation and outlook. But if you ever find things are just getting too much, don't be afraid to talk to your GP. They will be able to take you through the options available to you and offer advice. And don't forget about the wealth of help and advice available via the online community – with myriad forums full of like-minded sufferers discussing various issues – which will help you on the path through this stage in your life to a new and more confident you.

Notes

....
....
....
....
....
....
....
....
....
....
....
....
....
....
....

If you're interested in finding out more about our books,
find us on Facebook at **Summersdale Publishers**
and follow us on Twitter at **@Summersdale**.

www.summersdale.com